SUPER EASY GASTRITIS
DIET AND RECIPES

"Simple Gastritis Diet and Delicious Recipes"

Anita F. MS RDN McCluskey

Copyright © 2024 by Anita F. MS, RDN.McCluskey

All rights reserved. No part of this publication may be reproduced, distributed, or transmitted in any form or by any means, including photocopying, recording, or other electronic or mechanical methods, without the prior written permission of the publisher, except in the case of brief quotations embodied in critical reviews and certain other noncommercial uses permitted by copyright law.

Legal notice: This book is protected by copyright law and is intended for personal use only. Without explicit permission from the publisher or author, you are prohibited from altering, distributing, selling, quoting, or paraphrasing any portion of the book's content.

Disclaimer

The recipes and information provided in this super easy gastritis diet and recipes are intended for educational and informational purposes only. It is not a substitute for professional medical advice, diagnosis, or treatment. Always seek the advice of your physician or other qualified health provider with any questions you may have regarding a medical condition. The author and publisher of this cookbook are not liable for any adverse effects or consequences resulting from the use of the information or recipes contained herein."

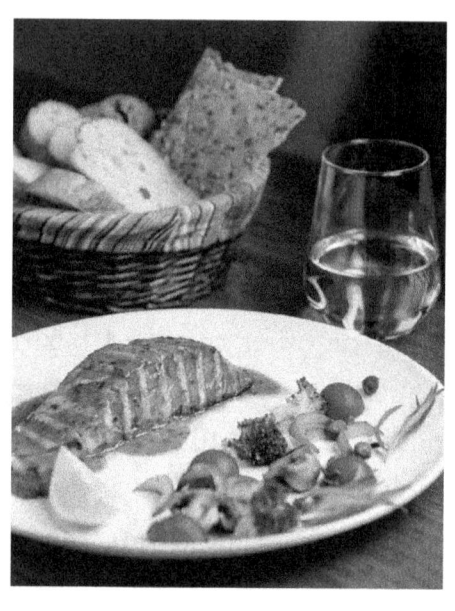

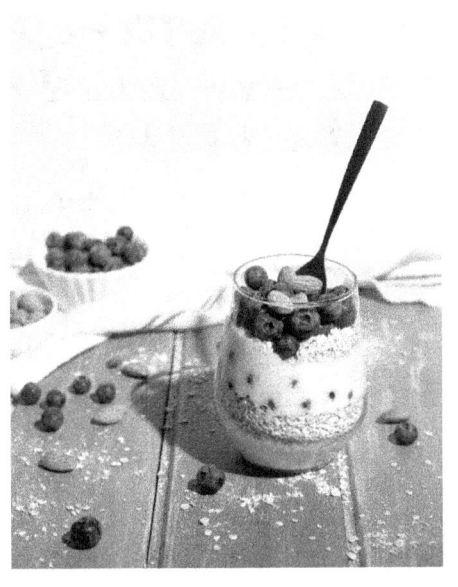

"Gastritis Mastery: The Ultimate Guide to Transforming from Novice to Pro with Special Hank's Expertise"

Welcome to "Gastritis Mastery," your roadmap to mastering gastritis diet and recipes with the guidance of Special Hank. This book is designed to help you progress from a novice to a highly skilled grandmaster in managing gastritis effortlessly. Let's embark on this journey together.

Gastritis Fundamentals:

1. Understand the basics: causes, symptoms, and triggers of gastritis.
2. Learn how diet impacts gastritis management and symptom alleviation.
3. Gain insights from Special Hank's personal experiences and expert advice.

2: Building Your Gastritis Diet Foundation

1. Establish a strong foundation with easy-to-follow dietary guidelines.
2. Stock your kitchen with gastritis-friendly essentials and alternatives.

3. Learn meal planning techniques to ensure balanced nutrition and symptom control.

3: Super Easy Gastritis diet and Recipes

1. Explore a variety of delicious and soothing recipes tailored for gastritis sufferers.
2. Follow Special Hank's favorite recipes, carefully crafted for taste and ease of preparation.
3. Discover cooking tips and techniques to enhance flavor without aggravating symptoms.

4: Advanced Strategies for Gastritis Mastery

1. Fine-tune your diet by identifying and avoiding trigger foods.
2. Incorporate stress management and lifestyle adjustments for optimal symptom control.
3. Learn from Special Hank's advanced tactics and expert insights for long-term gastritis management.

Progressing with Special Hank to Grandmaster Level

- Track your progress and celebrate milestones along the way.
- Adapt recipes and dietary strategies to suit your individual preferences and needs.
- Harness Special Hank's expertise to confidently navigate challenges and setbacks.

Conclusion:

Congratulations on completing your journey from novice to pro in managing gastritis with the help of Special Hank. Armed with the knowledge and skills acquired from this book, you are now equipped to become a highly skilled grandmaster in gastritis management. Here's to your continued health and success!

PREFACE

Welcome to "Super Easy Gastritis Diet and Recipes"! This book is designed to be your ultimate guide to managing gastritis symptoms through simple dietary adjustments and delicious recipes. Whether you're newly diagnosed or seeking ways to alleviate discomfort, you'll find practical tips, meal plans, and mouthwatering dishes tailored to soothe your stomach and nourish your body. Let this book be your companion on the journey to better digestive health.

TABLE OF CONTENT

"Gastritis Mastery: The Ultimate Guide to Transforming from Novice to Pro with Special Hank's Expertise"

PREFACE

Introduction

Chapter 1: Grasping Gastritis

Chapter 2: Understanding the Significance of Dietary Choices in Gastritis Management

Chapter 3: Establishing a Kitchen Suitable for Gastritis

Chapter 4: Simple Gastritis-Friendly Recipes

Chapter 5: Meal Plans for Gastritis Management

Chapter 6: Guidelines for Eating Out with Gastritis

Chapter 7: Coping with Stress and Gastritis

Chapter 8: Sustaining Motivation and Consistency

"Super Easy Gastritis Diet and Recipes: A 30-Day Meal Plan for Soothing Your Stomach"

Conclusion:

Introduction

Welcome to "Super Easy Gastritis Diet and Recipes," your go-to guide for managing gastritis with simple dietary adjustments and tasty recipes. Whether you're new to dealing with gastritis or seeking relief from symptoms, this book provides the knowledge and recipes to support your digestive health.

Gastritis, marked by stomach lining inflammation, can disrupt daily life. But with the right diet, you can take charge of your gastritis and enhance your well-being. Explore the basics of gastritis, its causes, symptoms, and triggers. Learn how food choices and lifestyle habits affect symptoms, empowering you to make informed decisions.

This book isn't just about limitations; it's about discovering flavorful, healing foods. From comforting soups to nutritious meals, our recipes are both delicious and easy to prepare, ensuring you enjoy your gastritis-friendly diet.

Find breakfast, lunch, and dinner ideas, along with tips for meal planning, grocery shopping, and dining out. With these resources, you'll successfully navigate your gastritis journey.

Embrace a gastritis-friendly diet with our recipes to manage symptoms, promote healing, and enhance your quality of life. Join us on the path to better digestive health and a happier you.

Chapter 1: Grasping Gastritis

Embark on an illuminating journey into gastrointestinal health with "Understanding Gastritis," an extensive handbook devoted to comprehending, handling, and averting gastritis. This section seamlessly merges medical knowledge with practical advice to empower readers in their pursuit of digestive wellness.

Commence with a thorough examination of the digestive system, unraveling the intricate connections among organs and functions vital for optimal digestion. Delve into the significance of the stomach lining and the delicate equilibrium of gastric acid production, laying the groundwork for grasping gastritis.

Explore the definition of gastritis, uncovering its origins, indications, and diagnostic methodologies. Through lucid explanations, unearth the myriad factors influencing gastritis, spanning from dietary patterns to bacterial infections such as Helicobacter pylori.

Furthermore, "Understanding Gastritis" furnishes actionable tactics for symptom management and nurturing gastric well-being. From dietary modifications to scientifically-backed treatments and holistic remedies, this section offers a tailored approach to tackling gastritis.

Enriched with captivating visuals, informative schematics, and real-world instances, Chapter 1 establishes a robust framework for navigating the intricacies of gastritis with assurance. Whether seeking relief from discomfort, preventing recurrence, or bolstering overall health, this chapter serves as an invaluable guide for effective gastritis care.

Understanding Gastritis:

Gastritis is a health condition characterized by inflammation or irritation of the stomach lining. This inflammation can occur suddenly, known as acute gastritis, or gradually over time, termed chronic gastritis. It can affect individuals of all ages and may lead to various symptoms and complications if not addressed.

Causes of Gastritis:

Several factors can cause gastritis, including:
1. Infection with Helicobacter pylori: This bacterium is a common cause of gastritis as it infects the stomach lining,
 leading to inflammation.

2. Regular use of nonsteroidal anti-inflammatory drugs (NSAIDs): Prolonged use of medications like aspirin and ibuprofen can irritate the stomach lining.

3. _Excessive alcohol consumption:_ Alcohol can irritate the stomach lining, increasing the risk of gastritis.

4. _Bile reflux:_ When bile flows back into the stomach, it can irritate the lining and cause inflammation.

5. _Autoimmune disorders:_
Autoimmune disorders, such as autoimmune gastritis, occur when the immune system erroneously targets the cells of the stomach lining, leading to inflammation and damage.

6. _Stress:_ While stress itself may not directly cause gastritis, it can exacerbate symptoms or trigger flare-ups.

Symptoms of Gastritis:
Symptoms of gastritis vary depending on its severity and type and may include:
1. Abdominal discomfort or pain, varying in intensity.
2. Nausea and vomiting, particularly after eating.

3. Indigestion, characterized by bloating, belching, and a feeling of fullness.
4. Loss of appetite, leading to weight loss or nutritional deficiencies.
5. Burning or gnawing sensation in the stomach's upper part.
6. Presence of blood in vomit or stool in severe cases.

Types of Gastritis:

Gastritis encompasses various types, such as:

1. Acute gastritis, which develops suddenly due to factors like NSAID use or bacterial infections.
2. Chronic gastritis, gradually developing over time and often caused by long-term inflammation or infections.
3. Erosive gastritis, resulting in stomach lining damage, potentially leading to ulcers or bleeding.
4. Autoimmune gastritis, where the immune system mistakenly attacks stomach lining cells, causing chronic inflammation.

Diagnosing Gastritis:

Healthcare providers diagnose gastritis through:
1. Medical history and physical examination to assess symptoms and potential risk factors.
2. Blood tests to identify underlying causes like H. pylori infection or anemia.
3. Stool tests to detect blood presence, indicating digestive tract bleeding.
4. Endoscopy, using a camera-equipped tube to examine the stomach lining for inflammation or damage.
5. Biopsy involves the collection of a small tissue sample during endoscopy for microscopic examination.

Understanding the causes, symptoms, types, and diagnostic approaches to gastritis enables individuals to manage their condition effectively and seek appropriate medical intervention when needed. Early detection and treatment can prevent complications and enhance overall health and well-being.

Chapter 2: Understanding the Significance of Dietary Choices in Gastritis Management

Gastritis, characterized by inflammation of the stomach lining, requires a comprehensive approach to treatment, with diet playing a pivotal role. Let's explore how dietary habits impact gastritis management, including foods to avoid, foods that offer relief, and the importance of lifestyle adjustments.

The Impact of Diet on Gastritis

Diet is crucial in managing gastritis as certain foods can either aggravate inflammation or aid in healing. Spicy, acidic, fatty, caffeinated, and alcoholic foods can irritate the stomach lining, worsening symptoms. Conversely, opting for bland, easily digestible foods can help alleviate discomfort and support the healing process.

Foods to Steer Clear of Gastritis

1. Spicy Fare: Steer clear of spicy foods like hot peppers and curry, as they can inflame the stomach lining.

2. Acidic Choices: Limit or avoid citrus fruits, tomatoes, and vinegar, as they can increase stomach acidity.

3. High-Fat Options: Cut back on fried foods, fatty meats, and rich desserts, as they can prolong inflammation.

4. Caffeine and Alcohol: Both can irritate the stomach lining and stimulate acid production, exacerbating gastritis symptoms.

Gastritis-Soothing Foods

1. Non-Acidic Fruits: Choose gentle options like bananas and apples for essential nutrients without stomach irritation.

2. Gentle Vegetables: Opt for cooked or steamed vegetables such as carrots and spinach for easy digestion.

3. Whole Grains: Incorporate fiber-rich whole grains like oats and brown rice to promote digestive health.

4. Lean Proteins: Include lean sources like poultry and tofu for essential amino acids minus excessive fat.

Embracing Lifestyle Changes

Beyond dietary adjustments, certain lifestyle changes complement gastritis management:

1. Stress Reduction: Practice stress-relieving activities like mindfulness and deep breathing to alleviate symptoms.

2. Consistent Eating: Opt for smaller, more frequent meals to minimize stomach acid production and discomfort.

3. _Adequate Hydration_: Stay well-hydrated throughout the day to support digestion.

4. _Avoid Smoking_: Quitting smoking or avoiding exposure to secondhand smoke is crucial for gastric health.

By adopting a gastritis-friendly diet and embracing lifestyle modifications, individuals can effectively manage symptoms and facilitate healing. Collaborating with healthcare professionals is key to developing a personalized treatment plan aligned with individual needs and preferences.

Chapter 3: Establishing a Kitchen Suitable for Gastritis

Crafting a gastritis-friendly kitchen entails more than merely selecting appropriate foods. It involves stocking your pantry with ingredients that are gentle on the stomach, ensuring you have essential kitchen tools, and becoming proficient in meal preparation techniques to facilitate healthy eating. Let's delve into the steps for creating a gastritis-friendly kitchen methodically.

Stocking Your Pantry

1. Whole Grains: Maintain a variety of whole grains like oats, brown rice, quinoa, and whole wheat pasta. These grains are stomach-friendly and offer vital nutrients and fiber.

2. Non-Acidic Fruits and Vegetables: Ensure you have non-acidic fruits such as bananas, apples, and melons, along with vegetables like carrots, spinach, and sweet potatoes. These options are easily digestible and packed with essential vitamins and minerals.

3. Lean Proteins: Opt for lean protein sources such as skinless poultry, fish, tofu, and legumes. These proteins are less likely to cause stomach irritation and supply crucial amino acids.

4. Low-Fat Dairy: Choose low-fat dairy products like yogurt, kefir, and lactose-free milk. These dairy options are gentler on the stomach and provide calcium for bone health.

5. Herbs and Spices: Utilize mild herbs and spices like ginger, turmeric, basil, and mint to enhance flavor without upsetting the stomach.

6. Healthy Fats: Incorporate sources of healthy fats such as olive oil, avocados, and nuts in moderation. These fats are less likely to cause inflammation and promote cardiovascular health.

7. Fiber-Rich Foods: Integrate high-fiber foods like chia seeds, flaxseeds, and psyllium husk to support digestive health and regular bowel movements.

Essential Kitchen Tools

1. Blender or Food Processor: These are handy for creating smoothies, pureeing soups, and preparing homemade sauces and dips.

2. Steamer Basket: A steamer basket allows you to cook vegetables gently without compromising their nutrients or texture.

3. Non-Stick Cookware: Non-stick cookware reduces the need for excessive fats and oils during cooking, making it gentler on the stomach.

4. Sharp Knives: Sharp knives facilitate safer and more efficient food preparation, enabling you to chop fruits, vegetables, and proteins with ease.

5. Measuring Cups and Spoons: Accurate measurement is crucial for following recipes and managing portion sizes effectively.

6. *Food Storage Containers*: Invest in a variety of food storage containers to store prepped ingredients and leftovers safely in the refrigerator or freezer.

Meal Prep Tips

1. *Plan Ahead*: Dedicate time each week to plan your meals and snacks, promoting healthier choices and reducing last-minute stress.

2. *Batch Cooking*: Prepare large quantities of grains, proteins, and vegetables in advance and portion them out for convenient meals throughout the week.

3. *Prep Ingredients*: Wash, chop, and portion out fruits, vegetables, and other ingredients ahead of time to streamline meal preparation.

4. *Label and Date*: Label and date your food containers to keep track of their contents and preparation dates.

5. Freeze Extras: If you've cooked more than needed, freeze surplus portions for future use, minimizing food waste and ensuring you always have gastritis-friendly options available.

By stocking your pantry with stomach-soothing ingredients, equipping yourself with essential kitchen tools, and mastering meal prep techniques, you can establish a gastritis-friendly kitchen that promotes digestive health and overall well-being. Experiment with various ingredients and recipes to discover what suits you best, and consider consulting a healthcare professional or registered dietitian for personalized guidance.

Chapter 4: Simple Gastritis-Friendly Recipes

Welcome to Chapter 4 of our gastritis-friendly recipe guide. Here, we present a variety of straightforward yet delightful recipes tailored to soothe and assist individuals dealing with gastritis. These recipes are carefully crafted to be gentle on the stomach while still offering delicious flavors and essential nutrients. Whether you're seeking relief from gastritis symptoms or simply in search of nourishing meal ideas, this chapter caters to all tastes and needs.

Breakfast Ideas:

1. Restorative Chicken Broth:

Restorative Chicken Broth boasts a long-standing history, revered for its healing qualities and delightful flavor, with roots tracing back centuries.

Traditionally, it involves simmering chicken bones, vegetables, herbs, and spices in water for extended periods, allowing the extraction of nutrients and creating a wholesome broth.

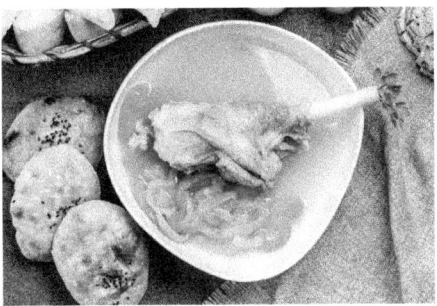

Ingredients:

- Chicken bones (best if organic)
- Water
- Vegetables (such as carrots, celery, onions)
- Herbs and spices (like parsley, thyme, bay leaves, and peppercorns)
- Optional: Salt

Preparation Time:

The preparation duration varies but typically lasts between 2 to 4 hours, depending on the desired depth of flavor and ingredient quantities.

Nutritional Value:

This broth is packed with collagen, gelatin, amino acids, and essential minerals like calcium, magnesium, and phosphorus. It maintains a low-calorie and low-fat profile, aiding in digestion. Furthermore, it aids in hydration, crucial for those with gastritis.

Tips for Gastritis Patients:

1. Low-Fat Variation: Trim excess fat from the broth to make it gentler on the stomach.

2. Gentle Cooking: Ensure a gentle simmer to prevent irritation to the stomach lining.

3. Thorough Straining: Filter the broth meticulously to eliminate any solid particles that might trigger discomfort.

4. Mild Seasoning: Opt for gentle spices and herbs, avoiding potent options like chili or garlic that may worsen gastritis symptoms.

5. Moderate Portions: Start with small servings and gradually increase as tolerated.

6. Observant Monitoring: Pay close attention to how your body reacts to the broth. Adjust ingredients or cooking times accordingly if discomfort arises.

7.Consultation for Supplements:
Seek advice from a healthcare professional regarding supplements that may compensate for any nutrients your diet lacks due to gastritis.

Restorative Chicken Broth not only acts as a soothing remedy for gastritis but also serves as a nutritious foundation for soups and various dishes, fostering overall well-being and contentment.

2. Ginger and Turmeric Infusion:
Golden milk, also known as ginger and turmeric infusion, boasts a long history in traditional medicine, particularly within Ayurveda. These ingredients, ginger and turmeric, revered for centuries, offer medicinal benefits. Ginger aids in digestion and reduces inflammation, while turmeric

contains curcumin, recognized for its potent antioxidant and anti-inflammatory properties.

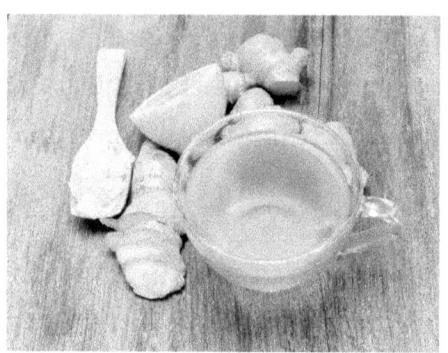

To prepare:
1. Peel and grate fresh ginger and turmeric roots (if using).
2. Combine them with milk in a saucepan.
3. Optionally, add spices like cinnamon, black pepper, or cardamom.
4. Simmer the mixture over medium heat for 5-10 minutes.
5. Strain it to remove the remnants.
6. Sweeten with honey, maple syrup, or stevia to taste.

Nutritional content varies based on milk type and sweetener. Nonetheless, both ingredients are low in calories and fat, rich in antioxidants, and possess anti-inflammatory qualities.

Gastritis tips:

1. Ginger and turmeric's anti-inflammatory properties can alleviate gastritis symptoms.
2. Fresh roots offer maximum potency, but powdered forms are effective too.
3. Limit sweeteners to avoid exacerbating symptoms.
4. Start with small amounts of sensitivity, gradually increasing as tolerated.
5. Consume warm rather than hot to avoid stomach irritation.

Incorporating golden milk into a gastritis-friendly diet can provide comfort and potential relief.

However, consulting a healthcare professional is advised, especially for those with underlying health concerns.

A comforting and warm tea infused with the healing properties of ginger and turmeric. This anti-inflammatory drink is perfect for settling an upset stomach and aiding digestion.

3. Mildly Seasoned Baked Fish:

Origin: Drawing from the rich culinary heritage of the Mediterranean, this dish has stood the test of time as a delectable and nutritious choice among seafood enthusiasts.

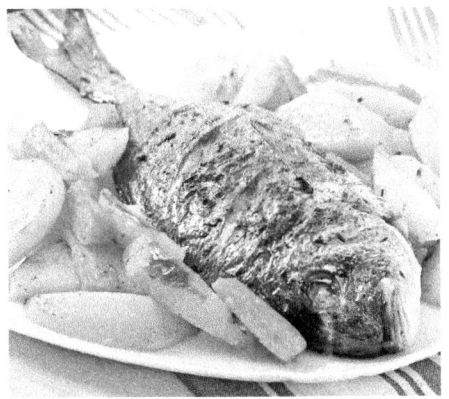

Ingredients:
1. Filets of white fish (like cod, haddock, or tilapia)
2. Olive oil
3. Lemon juice
4. Minced garlic
5. Paprika
6. Salt and pepper, to taste
7. Fresh herbs (such as parsley or dill) for garnish

Preparation Time: Takes around 25-30 minutes

Nutritional Value (per serving):

1. Calories: Caloric content varies based on fish type and portion size, typically ranging from 150 to 200 calories

2. Protein: A rich source, offering between 20-25 grams per serving

3. Healthy fats from olive oil

4. Low carbohydrate content

Gastritis-Friendly Tips :

1. Select gentle seasonings to avoid upsetting the stomach.
2. Opt for fresh, premium ingredients to minimize potential irritants.
3. Choose lean white fish, known for its easier digestibility.
4. Ensure careful cooking to preserve moisture and tenderness, which can be gentler on sensitive stomachs.

5.Accompany with steamed vegetables or a simple salad for a well-rounded, stomach-friendly meal.

This dish provides a delicate yet flavorful option that's well-suited for individuals managing gastritis.

4. Wholesome Mashed Sweet Potatoes:

Here's a crafted history for the Wholesome Mashed Sweet Potatoes recipe:

"Wholesome Mashed Sweet Potatoes have a rich history dating back centuries, originating in regions where sweet potatoes were cultivated abundantly. Initially cherished for their natural sweetness and versatility, sweet potatoes became a staple in many cuisines worldwide.

However, it wasn't until the modern era that the idea of mashing sweet potatoes gained widespread popularity. With the growing interest in healthier alternatives to traditional mashed potatoes, chefs and home cooks began experimenting with sweet potatoes as a nutritious and flavorful alternative.

Over time, various recipes emerged, each adding its own twist to the classic dish. Some incorporated butter and milk for added richness, while others emphasized the natural sweetness of the sweet potatoes with minimal seasoning.

In recent years, the Wholesome Mashed Sweet Potatoes recipe has gained traction among health-conscious individuals and those with dietary restrictions. With its simple preparation and nutritious profile, it has become a go-to side dish for family dinners, holiday gatherings, and special occasions.

As awareness of digestive health issues like gastritis has increased, the recipe has been adapted to accommodate sensitive stomachs. By omitting ingredients that may aggravate gastric symptoms and focusing on gentle seasonings, this dish continues to provide comfort and nourishment to a diverse range of individuals.

Today, Wholesome Mashed Sweet Potatoes remain a beloved dish cherished not only for its taste but also for its health benefits and adaptability to various dietary needs."

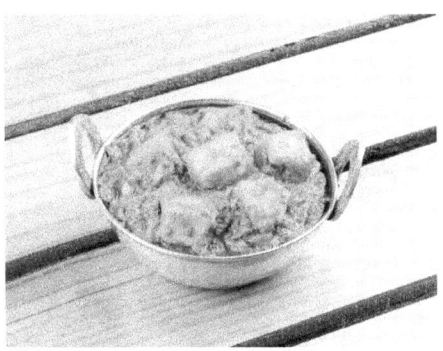

Wholesome Mashed Sweet Potatoes

Ingredients:

4 medium-sized sweet potatoes
2 tablespoons of unsalted butter or olive oil
1/4 cup of milk (you can use almond milk or any dairy-free alternative)
Salt and pepper to taste
Optional: a dash of cinnamon or nutmeg for added flavor

Preparation Time:

Prep: 10 minutes
Cook: 30 minutes
Total: 40 minutes

Instructions:

Preheat your oven to 400°F (200°C).
Wash the sweet potatoes thoroughly and prick each one several times with a fork.
Place the sweet potatoes on a baking sheet lined with parchment paper and bake for 30-40 minutes, or until they are tender and can be easily pierced with a fork.
Once the sweet potatoes are cooked, allow them to cool slightly before handling.
Peel the skin off the sweet potatoes and place the flesh into a mixing bowl.
Add the butter or olive oil, milk, salt, and pepper to the bowl.
Mash everything together using a potato masher or fork until you reach your desired consistency. If you

prefer smoother mashed sweet potatoes, you can use a hand blender.

Taste and adjust seasoning if necessary. If you like, add a dash of cinnamon or nutmeg for extra flavor. Serve hot and enjoy!

Nutritional Value (per serving, approximately 1/2 cup):

Calories: 150
Total Fat: 4g
Saturated Fat: 2g
Cholesterol: 10mg
Sodium: 85mg
Total Carbohydrates: 27g
Dietary Fiber: 4g
Sugars: 7g
Protein: 2g

Tips for Gastritis:

Sweet potatoes are generally well-tolerated by individuals with gastritis due to their low acidity and mild flavor.

To make this dish even more gentle on the stomach, you can omit the butter and use olive oil instead.

Avoid adding too much salt or spices, as they can irritate the stomach lining. Stick to mild seasonings like salt and pepper.

It's best to consume mashed sweet potatoes warm or at room temperature, as hot temperatures can sometimes aggravate gastritis symptoms.

If you're experiencing a flare-up of gastritis, consider consulting with a healthcare professional for personalized dietary advice.

Velvety and nutritious mashed sweet potatoes, subtly seasoned and gentle on the digestive system. Loaded with vitamins and fiber, this side dish provides both comfort and nourishment.

5. Turkey Meatballs:

Origin of Turkey Meatballs:

Turkey meatballs have a long history, originating from Turkish cuisine. They're a twist on traditional meatballs, swapping beef or pork for ground turkey. They've become popular worldwide for their leaner meat and healthier profile.

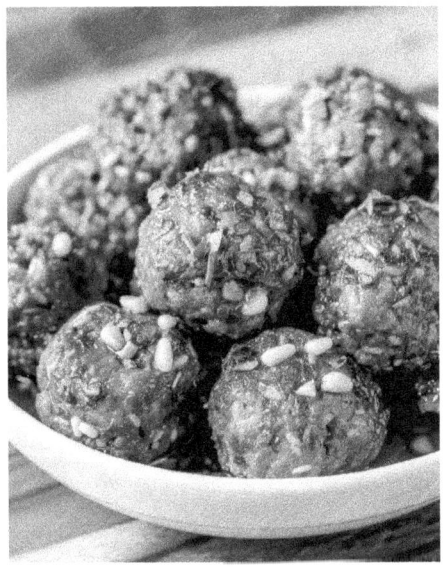

Ingredients:

1. 1 pound ground turkey
2. 1/2 cup breadcrumbs
3. 1/4 cup grated Parmesan cheese
4. 1/4 cup chopped parsley
5. 1 egg

6. 2 cloves garlic, minced
7. 1/2 teaspoon salt
8. 1/4 teaspoon black pepper
9. Olive oil (for cooking)

Preparation Time:

Prepping turkey meatballs takes about 15-20 minutes, and they cook in roughly 15-20 minutes, depending on size.

Nutritional Value:

Turkey meatballs are a healthier option than traditional ones, boasting lower fat and calorie content. Here's an approximate nutritional breakdown per serving (4 meatballs):

- Calories: 200
- Protein: 20g
- Fat: 10g
- Carbohydrates: 6g
- Fiber: 1g

Gastritis-Friendly Tips:

For those with gastritis or sensitive stomachs, here are some helpful suggestions:

1. Opt for lean ground turkey to reduce fat, which can be gentler on the stomach.

2. Skip spicy ingredients like chili powder or hot sauce, as they can worsen gastritis symptoms.

3. Choose low-fat cooking methods such as baking or grilling instead of frying.

4. Use whole wheat breadcrumbs or gluten-free alternatives if gluten is an issue.

5. Add grated carrots or zucchini to the mix for extra moisture and nutrients without irritating the stomach lining.

Following these tips allows you to enjoy tasty turkey meatballs while keeping gastritis symptoms in check.

Mix ground turkey with breadcrumbs, egg, garlic, and seasoning. Bake and serve with pasta and marinara sauce.

6. Honeyed Oatmeal with Banana:

Evolution of Honeyed Oatmeal with Banana:

The cherished morning meal of honeyed oatmeal with banana has roots in the timeless tradition of blending nourishing oats with the innate sweetness of bananas and honey. Oats, celebrated for centuries for their nutritional richness and adaptability, form the hearty base of this dish. Bananas, renowned for their potassium abundance and creamy texture, harmonize seamlessly with the robust oats. The introduction of honey provides a delicate sweetness, elevating the overall flavor experience.

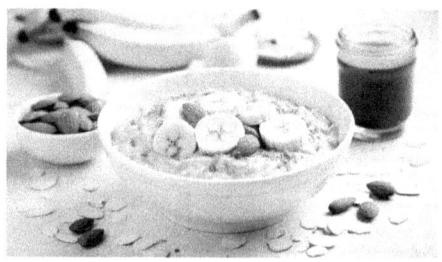

Ingredients:

- Rolled oats
- Liquid base: water or milk (dairy or plant-based)
- Ripe bananas
- Honey
- Optional toppings: nuts, seeds, cinnamon

Preparation Time:
Typically, preparation spans 10-15 minutes.

Nutritional Composition:

1. Oats: Abundant in fiber, protein, and an array of essential vitamins and minerals such as manganese, phosphorus, and magnesium. Oats are celebrated for their cardiovascular benefits and digestive support.

2. Bananas: Brimming with potassium, vitamin C, and vitamin B6, bananas offer swift energy and contribute to digestive wellness.

3. Honey: While imparting sweetness, honey also boasts antioxidants and potential antibacterial properties. However, its consumption should be moderated due to its high sugar content.

Gastritis-friendly Suggestions:
1. Opt for ripe bananas: Ripe bananas are gentler on the stomach and easier to digest compared to their unripe counterparts.
2. Thoroughly cooked oats: Ensuring oats are fully cooked enhances their digestibility, diminishing the likelihood of stomach irritation.
3. Select low-acid sweeteners: While honey provides sweetness, its consumption should be limited for individuals with gastritis to mitigate potential symptom exacerbation.

Consider utilizing minimal amounts of honey or exploring alternatives like maple syrup.
4. Experiment with toppings: Incorporating nuts or seeds into the oatmeal offers additional nutrients and textures without aggravating gastritis symptoms. Cinnamon serves as a flavorful option that may possess anti-inflammatory properties.

By adhering to these guidelines and indulging in honeyed oatmeal with banana in moderation, one can relish a delectable and nutritious breakfast while remaining attentive to gastritis concerns.

A comforting and filling breakfast choice that's easy on the stomach. Smooth oatmeal topped with ripe banana slices and a hint of honey delivers sustained energy without discomfort.

7. Lightly Steamed Vegetables:

History:

Lightly steamed vegetables have been a dietary staple for centuries. Originating in ancient China, steaming has long been valued for its ability to preserve the natural flavors and nutrients of vegetables, spreading to various cultures over time.

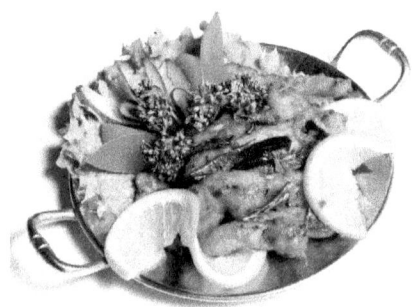

Ingredients:

Lightly steamed vegetables typically include a variety such as broccoli, carrots, cauliflower, green beans, zucchini, and bell peppers. You'll also need water for steaming and optional seasonings like salt, pepper, herbs, or lemon juice for added flavor.

Preparation Time:

The preparation time for lightly steamed vegetables varies depending on the types and quantities being cooked. Generally, it takes about 5-10 minutes to chop the vegetables and another 5-10 minutes to steam them.

Nutritional Value:

Lightly steamed vegetables retain more nutrients compared to boiling or frying methods. They are packed with essential vitamins, minerals, fiber, and antioxidants, including Vitamin C, Vitamin K, folate, potassium, and fiber.

Tips for Gastritis:

For individuals with gastritis or sensitive stomachs, lightly steamed vegetables can be a gentle option. Here are some tips to consider:

1. Opt for easily digestible vegetables like carrots, zucchini, and green beans.
2. Steam the vegetables until tender but still slightly crisp to prevent irritation to the stomach lining.
3. Limit the use of seasoning to avoid triggering gastritis symptoms.
4. Consume smaller, more frequent servings of steamed vegetables to avoid overloading the stomach.
5. If certain vegetables worsen your gastritis symptoms, try alternative options that are better tolerated.

Enjoy incorporating lightly steamed vegetables into your diet for their nutritious and soothing benefits!

A vibrant assortment of steamed vegetables, delicately seasoned and brimming with essential nutrients. This straightforward side dish is stomach-friendly while offering a satisfying crunch and lively flavors.

8. Smoothie Bowl:

Smoothie bowls have surged in popularity recently, combining fruits, veggies, and other nutritious elements into a visually enticing dish. Originating from the traditional smoothie, this trend took off in the early 2010s, particularly on platforms like Instagram, where users flaunted their creatively adorned bowls with assorted toppings.

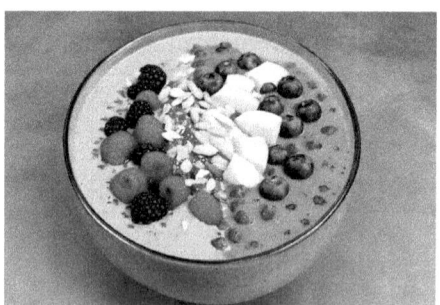

Ingredients:

Ingredients typically include a base of frozen fruits like bananas or berries, supplemented by non-dairy milk or yogurt. Additional fruits such as kiwi or pineapple, and vegetables like spinach or kale, contribute to flavor and nutrients. Protein options like protein powders or nut butter are often added, while toppings range from granola and nuts to seeds and shredded coconut.

Preparation Time:

Preparation usually takes 5-10 minutes, depending on ingredient prep. Smoothie bowls offer a rich blend of carbs, proteins, fats, vitamins, and minerals, but caution is advised regarding portion sizes and added sugars, especially for those with gastritis. Opting for low-acid fruits and non-acidic dairy substitutes can be beneficial.

Nutritional Value:

Smoothie bowls usually include an assortment of ingredients like fruits, vegetables, nuts, seeds, and liquid bases such as milk or yogurt. Their nutritional content can differ depending on the ingredients and amounts used, but they typically offer a wealth of vitamins, minerals, fiber, and antioxidants. Important nutrients like vitamin C, potassium, calcium, and beneficial fats are commonly found in smoothie bowls. For a detailed nutritional breakdown, the specific ingredients in your smoothie bowl would need to be specified.

Tips for Gastritis:
For those with gastritis, choosing fruits like bananas and melons over citrus fruits, avoiding spicy additions, and moderating fiber intake are recommended. Probiotic-rich ingredients like yogurt can also aid in gut health. With mindful ingredient choices and moderation, individuals with gastritis can still enjoy the nutritional benefits of smoothie bowls.

9. Yogurt Parfait:
The yogurt parfait boasts a rich history, originating in France before gaining global popularity as a go-to breakfast and snack. Comprising layers of yogurt, fruit, and granola, it offers a delightful blend of tastes and textures.

Historical Background:

The yogurt parfait's roots can be traced back to France, where it was dubbed "parfait aux fruits" or "perfect fruit." Its reputation as a wholesome and convenient morning meal surged in the United States during the latter half of the 20th century.

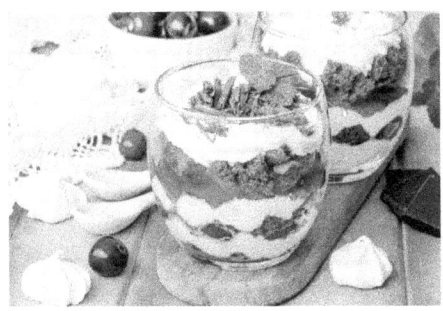

Ingredients:
1. Yogurt (options include Greek or regular yogurt)
2. Fresh fruits (like berries, bananas, or mango)
3. Granola or nuts
4. Optional: sweeteners such as honey or maple syrup

Preparation Time:

Crafting a yogurt parfait typically takes around 5-10 minutes, depending on the complexity of layering and ingredient selection.

Nutritional Composition:

The nutritional profile of a yogurt parfait varies depending on the chosen ingredients. Generally, it offers a balanced mix of protein from yogurt, fiber from fruits and granola, and essential vitamins and minerals. However, caution is advised regarding added sugars found in flavored yogurts and sweetened granola.

Gastritis-Friendly Tips:

For individuals managing gastritis, selecting stomach-friendly ingredients is crucial. Consider these suggestions:

1. Opt for low-fat or non-fat yogurt to minimize stomach irritation.
2. Prioritize ripe, soft fruits like bananas or cooked options over acidic varieties such as citrus fruits, which can exacerbate symptoms.
3. Choose plain yogurt over flavored alternatives to avoid artificial additives and excess sugars.

4. Moderation is key when adding granola or nuts, especially if they trigger discomfort.
5. Experiment with different toppings and textures to find what suits your stomach best.

Indulge in your yogurt parfait as a delightful and stomach-soothing treat!

Lunch Recipes:

1. Quinoa Salad:

Quinoa Salad has a long history, originating in the Andean region of South America, where it was a dietary staple for indigenous peoples like the Incas. Cultivated primarily in the Andes Mountains of Bolivia, Peru, and Ecuador, quinoa has gained global popularity in recent years due to its health benefits and culinary versatility.

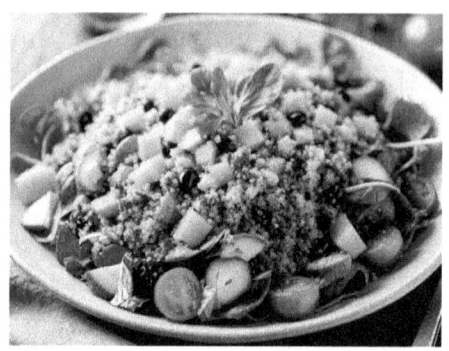

Ingredients for a standard Quinoa Salad typically include:

- **_Vegetables_:** Such as cherry tomatoes, cucumbers, bell peppers, red onions, and avocado.
- **_Greens_:** Options include spinach, kale, or arugula.
- **_Protein_:** Choices range from chickpeas, black beans, and tofu, to grilled chicken.
- **_Dressing_:** Typically a basic vinaigrette made with olive oil, lemon juice or vinegar, garlic, and herbs.

Preparation Time

Preparation time for Quinoa Salad varies depending on factors like ingredient choice and whether the quinoa is cooked from scratch. Typically, cooking quinoa takes 20-30 minutes, while chopping vegetables and preparing the dressing adds another 10-15 minutes, totaling roughly 30-45 minutes.

Nutritional Composition:
Nutritionally, quinoa is rich in protein, fiber, vitamins, and minerals, making it a valuable addition to any diet. Being gluten-free, it's also suitable for those with gluten intolerance or celiac disease.

For individuals with gastritis or sensitive stomachs, some considerations include:

1. Ensuring thorough cooking and rinsing of quinoa to remove saponins, which can irritate the stomach lining.
2. Avoid spicy or acidic ingredients in dressings, as they may worsen gastritis symptoms.
3. Opting for easily digestible vegetables and proteins, like cooked veggies and lean proteins such as tofu or grilled chicken.

4. Incorporating soothing ingredients like cucumber or avocado to help alleviate stomach inflammation.
5. Controlling portion sizes to prevent overwhelming the digestive system.

By adhering to these guidelines and tailoring ingredients to individual dietary needs, Quinoa Salad can offer a tasty and nourishing option for those managing gastritis or sensitive stomachs.

3. Tuna Salad Wrap origins:

Tuna salad wraps have emerged as a popular choice for a convenient and nutritious meal. While the idea of wrapping ingredients in soft tortillas or flatbreads has historical roots, the modern version of the tuna salad wrap likely gained popularity in the mid to late 20th century, reflecting the growing interest in portable foods.

Ingredients:

- Canned tuna
- Light mayonnaise or Greek yogurt
- Chopped celery
- Chopped onion
- Chopped pickles or relish
- Salt and pepper to taste
- Lettuce leaves
- Whole grain or spinach tortillas

Preparation Time:

- Takes approximately 10-15 minutes to prepare.

Nutritional Value:

1. Tuna provides protein, omega-3 fatty acids, and essential vitamins and minerals like vitamin D and selenium.
2. Light mayonnaise or Greek yogurt contributes creaminess and healthy fats or protein.
3. Vegetables such as celery, onion, and pickles offer flavor, fiber, and essential nutrients.

4. Whole grain or spinach tortillas provide complex carbohydrates, fiber, and additional vitamins and minerals.

Gastritis-Friendly Tips:
- Opt for light mayonnaise or Greek yogurt to reduce fat content, which can worsen gastritis symptoms.
- Choose low-sodium canned tuna to minimize salt intake, as excessive salt can irritate the stomach lining.
- Avoid spicy seasonings, onion, and garlic, which may trigger discomfort for those with gastritis.
- Select whole grain or spinach tortillas for added fiber, promoting digestive health and easing gastritis symptoms.
- If raw vegetables are harsh on your stomach, lightly cook them before adding to the wrap.

Enjoy your tasty and stomach-friendly tuna salad wrap!

Dinner Options:

1. Baked Salmon history:

Baked salmon has been a culinary tradition for centuries, likely originating alongside the discovery of fire for cooking.

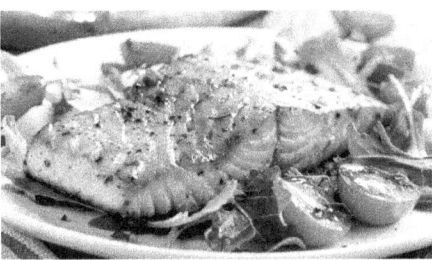

Ingredients:

To prepare baked salmon, you'll need salmon filets, olive oil, lemon slices, salt, pepper, and optional herbs like dill, parsley, or thyme.

Preparation Time:

Expect to spend around 20 to 30 minutes preparing baked salmon, depending on the recipe and filet thickness.

Nutritional Value:

A 3-ounce (85-gram) serving of baked salmon provides about 177 calories, 23 grams of protein, 9 grams of fat, and 1.5 grams of omega-3 fatty acids. It's also rich in vitamins D and B.

Tips for Gastritis:

For those with gastritis, it's important to prepare baked salmon gently on the stomach. Choose fresh salmon, go easy on heavy sauces and spices, use olive oil sparingly, cook thoroughly but avoid overcooking, consider marinating in a mild citrus-based marinade, and pair with cooked vegetables or a simple salad for a balanced, stomach-friendly meal.

2. Vegetable Soup History

Vegetable soup has been a culinary favorite for ages, appearing in various forms across different cultures worldwide. Its roots can be traced back to ancient civilizations, where people simmered vegetables in water or broth to craft a wholesome meal. Throughout history, culinary traditions have adapted the recipe to reflect local tastes and ingredients. Today, vegetable soup endures as a beloved dish cherished for its simplicity, adaptability, and healthful qualities.

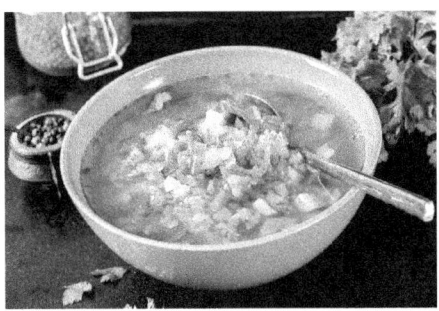

Ingredients:

1. An array of vegetables (like carrots, celery, onions, potatoes, tomatoes, bell peppers, spinach, and kale)
2. Broth (vegetable broth for vegetarians, or chicken/beef broth for added richness)
3. Herbs and spices (such as garlic, thyme, bay leaves, parsley, salt, and pepper)
4. Olive oil (for sautéing vegetables)
5. Optional protein (such as beans, lentils, or tofu)

Preparation Time:

The preparation duration for vegetable soup varies depending on the recipe and cooking method. On average, it typically takes around 30-45 minutes to prepare and cook vegetable soup, although certain recipes may require longer simmering periods to enhance flavor.

Nutritional Value:

Vegetable soup boasts an abundance of vital nutrients, making it a nourishing and calorie-conscious meal option. Bursting with vitamins, minerals, and antioxidants from a diverse mix of vegetables, it's also high in fiber, which aids digestion and promotes satiety. By opting for a low-sodium broth and minimizing added fats, vegetable soup emerges as a heart-friendly choice.

Tips for Gastritis:

For those with gastritis or sensitive stomachs, consider these guidelines when making vegetable soup:

1. Prioritize easily digestible vegetables, favoring softer options like carrots, potatoes, and squash, while steering clear of spicy or acidic ingredients like onions, tomatoes, and hot peppers.

2. Opt for a low-fat or fat-free broth to minimize the risk of exacerbating gastritis symptoms, and refrain from excessive use of oil or butter.

3. Ensure thorough cooking of vegetables until they're soft and easily digestible, as raw or undercooked vegetables may be harsh on the stomach.

4. Exercise moderation with seasoning; while herbs and spices enhance flavor, be cautious with quantities, particularly if certain spices tend to trigger gastritis symptoms.

5. Begin with small servings to gauge how your stomach reacts, gradually increasing portion sizes as tolerated.

By adhering to these recommendations and selecting gentle ingredients, vegetable soup can offer a comforting and nourishing option for individuals with gastritis.

Snacks and Desserts

1. Greek Yogurt with Honey historical background:

In ancient Greece, yogurt was a dietary staple, while honey held significant cultural importance as the "nectar of the gods." The combination of these two ingredients created a delightful and nourishing treat enjoyed for centuries. Greek yogurt's thick, creamy texture complements the natural sweetness of honey, resulting in a harmonious blend of flavors cherished by the Greeks throughout history.

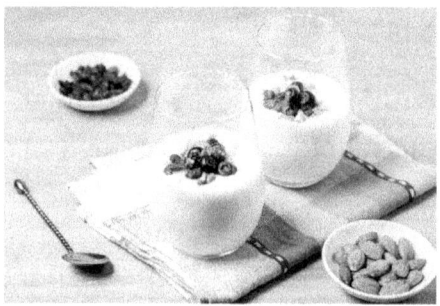

Ingredients:

Greek yogurt, renowned for its dense consistency achieved through straining, offers a rich source of protein, calcium, probiotics, and various nutrients. Meanwhile, honey, celebrated for its antioxidant and antimicrobial properties, serves as a natural sweetener, enhancing the flavor profile of the yogurt.

Preparation Time:
Crafting Greek yogurt with honey is a swift and straightforward process, typically requiring just five minutes to gather and blend the ingredients seamlessly.

Nutritional Profile:
Greek yogurt boasts high protein content alongside essential nutrients like calcium and probiotics crucial for gut health. Honey, while primarily comprising sugars, contains trace vitamins, minerals, and antioxidants.

Gastritis-Friendly Tips:

For individuals managing gastritis, selecting low-fat or fat-free Greek yogurt is advisable to minimize potential discomfort. Choosing raw, unprocessed honey may also be gentler on the stomach compared to processed alternatives. Moderation is key when enjoying Greek yogurt with honey, paying close attention to personal tolerance levels. Should any adverse reactions occur, seeking guidance from a healthcare professional is recommended for tailored advice.

Enjoy plain Greek yogurt with a drizzle of honey for a creamy snack.

2. Apple Slices with Almond Butter origin:

Apple slices paired with almond butter emerged as a popular, nutritious snack in recent years, driven by the growing interest in healthy eating and the rise of almond butter as a wholesome spread alternative.

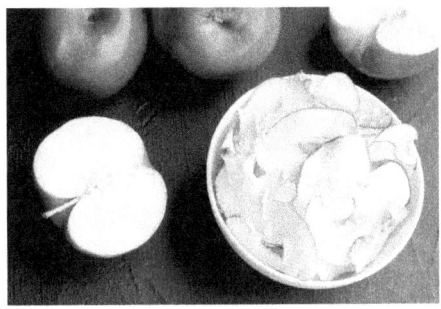

Ingredients:
- 1-2 crisp, sweet apples such as Gala or Fuji
- Natural, unsweetened almond butter

Preparation Time:
Preparation typically takes only 5-10 minutes, depending on the desired serving size.

Nutritional Benefits:
1. Apples provide fiber, vitamin C, and antioxidants, aiding in satiety and overall health.
2. Almond butter offers healthy fats, protein, vitamin E, magnesium, and fiber, promoting heart health and sustained energy.

Gastritis-Friendly Tips:

For those with gastritis or sensitive stomachs:

1. Choose softer, ripe apples to reduce stomach irritation.
2. Select almond butter free of added oils or sugars to avoid exacerbating symptoms.
3. Apply a thin layer of almond butter on each slice to moderate fat intake.
4. If raw apples are problematic, lightly steam or bake them before adding almond butter for easier digestion.

By incorporating these suggestions, individuals can savor the delightful combination of apple slices with almond butter while effectively managing gastritis symptoms.

3. Chia Seed Pudding:

Chia seed pudding boasts a rich history tracing back to ancient civilizations such as the Aztecs and Mayans, who revered chia seeds for their nutritional value. These seeds were a dietary staple in Central America, with Aztec warriors purportedly consuming them for sustained energy in battles. Despite their significance, chia seeds waned in popularity after the Spanish conquest. However, in recent times, they've seen a resurgence due to their nutritional richness and adaptability in recipes like chia seed pudding.

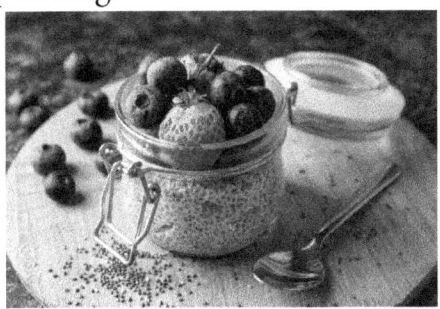

The ingredients typically include chia seeds, a liquid base like almond or coconut milk, optional sweeteners such as honey or maple syrup, and flavorings like vanilla extract or cocoa powder. While the preparation time for mixing these ingredients is short, the pudding requires several hours of refrigeration for the chia seeds to absorb the liquid and attain a pudding-like texture.

In terms of nutrition, chia seeds are packed with omega-3 fatty acids, fiber, protein, antioxidants, vitamins, and minerals, notably featuring high levels of alpha-linolenic acid beneficial for heart health. Moreover, they are gluten-free and easily digestible, making chia seed pudding a nutritious option for snacks or breakfast, offering sustained energy and satiety.

For individuals dealing with gastritis or sensitive stomachs, it's crucial to prepare chia seed pudding with ingredients that won't aggravate symptoms. Opting for low-acid liquids like almond or coconut milk over dairy, using natural sweeteners in moderation, avoiding acidic fruits or flavorings, starting with small portions, and seeking medical advice if discomfort persists are advisable steps for gastritis management.

Conclusion:
Chapter 4 presents a selection of gastritis-friendly recipes aimed at offering comfort, nourishment, and relief to those managing gastritis. With an emphasis on gentle ingredients and soothing flavors, these recipes allow for the enjoyment of delicious meals without worsening symptoms. Whether you're craving a revitalizing broth, a comforting tea, or a fulfilling main course, this chapter provides

simple yet flavorful options to support your health and well-being.

Chapter 5: Meal Plans for Gastritis Management

In the fifth chapter of our comprehensive gastritis management guide, we present practical meal plans tailored to alleviate symptoms and enhance digestive health. Gastritis, marked by inflammation of the stomach lining, necessitates careful dietary choices to minimize discomfort and aid in recovery. Each meal plan is crafted to strike a balance between nutrient-rich foods and the avoidance of triggers that could worsen symptoms.

Explanation of Meal Plan 2:

This meal plan prioritizes lean proteins, whole grains, and abundant fruits and vegetables to support digestive health. Turkey, tofu, and eggs provide easily digestible proteins, while avocado and olive oil contribute healthy fats to soothe the stomach lining. Fiber-rich whole grains like brown rice and quinoa promote digestive regularity, and colorful fruits and vegetables supply essential vitamins and minerals. Snacks like cottage cheese and peaches offer a delightful and nutritious option between meals. Overall, this meal plan is designed to alleviate inflammation and facilitate healing for individuals managing gastritis.

Gastritis management is supported by a well-rounded diet. Below are sample meal plans designed to soothe the stomach and aid in healing.

Meal Plan 1:

Breakfast:

- Start the day with oatmeal topped with sliced banana and a sprinkle of ground flaxseeds, accompanied by herbal tea or water.

Lunch:

- Enjoy a lunch of grilled chicken breast with a side of steamed vegetables like carrots, broccoli, and zucchini, paired with brown rice or quinoa. Complete the meal with a mixed green salad dressed with olive oil and lemon.

Snack:

- Opt for a light snack of plain yogurt with honey and a handful of almonds.

Dinner:

- Conclude the day with baked salmon served alongside roasted sweet potatoes and steamed asparagus, complemented by a whole grain roll.

Meal Plan 2:

Breakfast:

- Kick off your morning with whole-grain toast topped with mashed avocado and poached eggs, accompanied by a refreshing green smoothie made from spinach, banana, and almond milk.

Lunch:

- For lunch, indulge in a turkey and avocado wrap with lettuce and tomato, alongside carrot sticks with hummus and slices of apple.

Snack:
- Treat yourself to cottage cheese paired with sliced peaches as a satisfying midday snack.

Dinner:
- Finish off the day with a nourishing dinner of stir-fried tofu with bell peppers and broccoli, served with brown rice and a mixed green salad dressed with balsamic vinaigrette.

Customizing Your Meal Plan

- Seek guidance from healthcare experts or a dietitian to adapt these plans to your specific dietary needs and tastes.

- Experiment with different foods to find what suits your stomach best.

- Pay attention to your body's signals and adjust portion sizes and meal frequency accordingly.

- Maintain a food journal to monitor how different foods impact your symptoms and make necessary changes.

These meal plans offer nutritious and enjoyable options while addressing gastritis symptoms. Remember to stay hydrated and include ample fruits, veggies, whole grains, lean proteins, and healthy fats in your diet for optimal recovery and overall health.

Chapter 6: Guidelines for Eating Out with Gastritis

For those dealing with gastritis, dining out can pose challenges due to menu options that might worsen symptoms. In this chapter, we offer thorough advice to navigate restaurant meals while effectively managing gastritis.

Strategies for Dining Out Safely:

1. Select Restaurants Wisely: Opt for establishments known for healthier choices, such as those prioritizing fresh ingredients and customizable meals. Avoid fast food joints and places with heavily processed offerings.

2. Pre-check the Menu: Before going out, review the menu online if available. Seek stomach-friendly options like grilled or steamed dishes, while steering clear of spicy, acidic, and oily foods.

3. Request Customizations: Feel free to ask servers for dish modifications to align with your dietary requirements. Request meals without added spices, sauces, or oils known to trigger gastritis symptoms.

4. Prioritize Lean Proteins and Veggies: Look for dishes featuring lean proteins like grilled chicken, fish, or tofu, paired with lightly cooked vegetables. These choices are generally gentler on the stomach.

5. Mind Portion Sizes: Large portions can overwhelm the stomach and exacerbate symptoms. Consider ordering smaller servings or sharing dishes to avoid overeating.

6. Avoid Trigger Foods: Stay away from known gastritis triggers such as spicy dishes, acidic sauces, fried items, and carbonated drinks. Opt for water or herbal tea instead of alcohol or sodas.

7. Eat Slowly and Mindfully: Take your time to enjoy each bite and chew thoroughly. Eating slowly aids digestion and helps prevent overeating, reducing the risk of discomfort.

8. Control Portions: Despite good intentions, it's easy to overindulge. Keep an eye on portion sizes and stop eating when you feel comfortably full to prevent gastric issues.

9. Carry Digestive Aids: Consider bringing antacids or digestive enzymes when dining out as a precautionary measure. These can help alleviate symptoms if you accidentally consume trigger foods.

10. Tune into Your Body: Listen to your body's signals. If discomfort or symptoms arise, pause eating and take a breather. Seek medical assistance if issues persist or worsen.

By adhering to these guidelines, individuals managing gastritis can dine out without sacrificing their digestive well-being. With thoughtful planning and mindful selections, eating out can remain an enjoyable experience while effectively managing gastritis.

Chapter 7: Coping with Stress and Gastritis

Understanding how stress affects gastritis symptoms is crucial for maintaining overall health. Here's a breakdown:

The Relationship Between Stress and Gastritis:

1. Making Sense of the Connection: While stress itself doesn't directly cause gastritis, it can aggravate symptoms and escalate inflammation in the stomach lining, leading to discomfort flare-ups.

2. Impact of Stress Hormones: Stress triggers the release of hormones like cortisol and adrenaline, disrupting digestion and boosting stomach acid production. This prolonged disruption can irritate the stomach lining, worsening gastritis symptoms.

3. Emotional Toll: Coping with gastritis symptoms can induce stress, creating a feedback loop where stress exacerbates symptoms, and symptoms, in turn, elevate stress levels.

Strategies for Stress Relief:

1. Deep Breathing Exercises: Practice deep breathing techniques to calm the mind and relax the body. Inhale deeply through the nose for four counts, hold for four counts, and exhale slowly through the mouth for four counts.

2. Mindfulness and Meditation: Integrate mindfulness or meditation practices into your daily regimen to reduce stress and foster relaxation. Focus on the present moment and let go of worries about the past or future.

3. Regular Physical Activity: Engage in consistent exercise to release endorphins, natural mood boosters. Activities like walking, yoga, and swimming are particularly effective for stress reduction.

4. Healthy Lifestyle Choices: Prioritize self-care activities like sufficient sleep, a balanced diet, and hydration. Nurturing your body aids in stress management and helps alleviate gastritis symptoms.

5. Seeking Support: Reach out to friends, family, or healthcare professionals for guidance and support. Sharing your feelings and concerns can alleviate stress and offer insight into managing gastritis.

Incorporating stress-relief techniques into your daily routine can mitigate stress's impact on gastritis symptoms and enhance your overall well-being. Remember, managing stress is a journey, so be patient as you discover what works best for you.

Chapter 8: Sustaining Motivation and Consistency

Chapter 8 delves into the timeless struggle humans have faced in maintaining motivation and consistency across different epochs. From ancient civilizations like Egypt, Mesopotamia, and China, where discipline was often intertwined with religious or philosophical beliefs, to the Renaissance era where figures like Leonardo da Vinci and Michelangelo showcased unwavering dedication in their pursuits, history is replete with examples of the importance of perseverance. The Industrial Revolution introduced new challenges as capitalism and modern work settings demanded sustained motivation amid repetitive tasks. In the 20th century, psychologists explored motivation through theories like Maslow's hierarchy of needs, Herzberg's two-factor theory, and Skinner's reinforcement theory. Despite the digital age's distractions, sustaining motivation remains pertinent, with technology offering both challenges and solutions. Chapter 8 would likely offer practical strategies drawn from history, psychology, and personal development to overcome obstacles and achieve lasting success.

Consistently staying motivated is crucial when managing gastritis and striving for better health. Here's how to stay committed:

Establishing Achievable Goals:

1. Be Precise: Set clear, reachable goals that are specific and measurable. Rather than saying, "I want to eat better," try setting a goal like, "I will incorporate a portion of vegetables with each meal."

2. Break it Down: Divide big goals into smaller, more manageable tasks to avoid feeling overwhelmed and to stay focused on progress.

3. Set Deadlines: Give yourself reasonable deadlines for achieving your goals. Allow enough time for meaningful changes without pressure.

4. Track Your Progress: Keep tabs on your achievements and milestones. This can boost motivation and show how far you've come.

Overcoming Hurdles:

1. Recognize Challenges: Identify potential obstacles and plan ways to overcome them, whether it's dealing with cravings or time constraints.

2. Stay Adaptable: Be open to adjusting your approach. If something isn't working, try a new strategy. Flexibility is key to long-term success.

3. Seek Support: Don't hesitate to ask for help from friends, family, or healthcare professionals. Support can make a significant difference.

4. Practice Self-Compassion: Be kind to yourself, especially during setbacks. Remember that progress isn't always linear, and it's okay to have tough days.

Celebrating Achievements:

1. Acknowledge Successes: Take time to celebrate even small accomplishments. Every step forward deserves recognition.

2. Reward Yourself: Treat yourself to something special as a reward for reaching milestones.

3. Share Your Progress: Share your successes with others to reinforce motivation and inspire them.

By setting realistic goals, overcoming challenges, and celebrating successes, you can maintain motivation and consistency on your journey to better health with gastritis. Remember to be patient with yourself and celebrate every step forward, no matter how small.

"Super Easy Gastritis Diet and Recipes: A 30-Day Meal Plan for Soothing Your Stomach"

Embark on a journey to soothe your stomach with our comprehensive 30-day meal plan designed specifically for those battling gastritis. This book offers a variety of delicious and easy-to-prepare recipes that are gentle on the stomach yet bursting with flavor. From comforting soups and broths to nourishing salads and light meals, each recipe is carefully crafted to alleviate symptoms and promote healing. With detailed meal plans, shopping lists, and helpful tips, managing gastritis has never been easier. Say goodbye to discomfort and hello to a happier, healthier stomach with "Super Easy Gastritis Diet and Recipes" by your side.

Week 1:

Day 1:
1. **_Breakfast_:** Banana and almond butter smoothie.
2. **_Snack_:** Rice cakes with avocado.
3. **_Lunch_:** Grilled chicken salad with mixed greens and olive oil dressing.
4. **_Snack_:** Greek yogurt with honey.
5. **_Dinner_:** Baked fish with steamed vegetables.

Day 2:
- **_Breakfast_:** Oatmeal with sliced strawberries.
- **_Snack_:** Almonds.
- **_Lunch_:** Turkey and hummus wrap with a side of carrot sticks.
- **_Snack_:** Apple slices with peanut butter.
- **_Dinner_:** Quinoa with roasted vegetables.

Day 3:
1. **_Breakfast_:** Whole grain toast with avocado.
2. **_Snack_:** Cottage cheese with pineapple.

3. **_Lunch:_** Lentil soup with a side of whole grain crackers.
4. **_Snack:_** Greek yogurt with granola.
5. **_Dinner:_** Grilled salmon with steamed asparagus.

Day 4:
1. **_Breakfast_**: Smoothie with spinach, banana, and almond milk.
2. **_Snack:_** Rice cakes with almond butter.
3. **_Lunch:_** Chicken and vegetable stir-fry with brown rice.
4. **_Snack:_** Mixed berries.
5. **_Dinner:_** Baked tofu with sautéed kale.

Day 5:
- **_Breakfast:_** Scrambled eggs with spinach and tomatoes.
- **_Snack:_** Carrot sticks with hummus.
- **_Lunch:_** Quinoa salad with cucumber, cherry tomatoes, and feta cheese.
- **_Snack:_** Greek yogurt with honey.
- **_Dinner:_** Turkey chili with a side of steamed broccoli.

Day 6:
- **_Breakfast:_** Greek yogurt with sliced peaches.
- **_Snack:_** Almonds.
- **_Lunch:_** Grilled chicken Caesar salad.
- **_Snack:_** Apple slices with almond butter.
- **_Dinner:_** Baked cod with roasted Brussels sprouts.

Day 7:
- **_Breakfast:_** Whole grain pancakes with fresh berries.
- **_Snack:_** Cottage cheese with pineapple.
- **_Lunch:_** Tuna salad lettuce wraps with cucumber slices.
- **_Snack:_** Rice cakes with avocado.
- **_Dinner:_** Vegetable stir-fry with tofu.

Week 2:

Day 8:
- **_Breakfast:_** Greek yogurt with berries and a sprinkle of granola.

- **_Lunch_:** Grilled chicken salad with mixed greens, cherry tomatoes, cucumber, and balsamic vinaigrette.
- **_Dinner_:** Baked salmon with roasted vegetables (such as broccoli, carrots, and bell peppers) and quinoa.

Day 9:

- **_Breakfast_:** Scrambled eggs with spinach and whole wheat toast.
- **_Lunch_:** Turkey and avocado wrap with whole grain tortilla, lettuce, and tomato.
- **_Dinner_:** Stir-fried tofu with mixed vegetables and brown rice.

Day 10:

- **_Breakfast_:** Overnight oats with almond milk, chia seeds, and sliced banana.
- **_Lunch_:** Quinoa salad with black beans, corn, diced bell peppers, and lime vinaigrette.
- **_Dinner_:** Spaghetti squash with marinara sauce and turkey meatballs.

Day 11:
- **_Breakfast_:** Smoothie with spinach, banana, almond milk, and protein powder.
- **_Lunch_:** Lentil soup with whole grain bread.
- **_Dinner_:** Grilled shrimp skewers with a side of steamed broccoli and quinoa.

Day 12:
- **_Breakfast_:** Whole grain toast with avocado slices and poached eggs.
- **_Lunch_:** Chicken Caesar salad with romaine lettuce, grilled chicken breast, Parmesan cheese, and Caesar dressing.
- **_Dinner_:** Vegetable stir-fry with tofu and brown rice.

Day 13
- **_Breakfast_:** Greek yogurt parfait with honey, sliced almonds, and diced peaches.
- **_Lunch_**: Quinoa and black bean stuffed bell peppers.
- **_Dinner_:** Baked cod with asparagus and wild rice.

Day 14:
- ***Breakfast:*** Veggie omelet with mushrooms, bell peppers, and spinach.
- ***Lunch:*** Tuna salad with mixed greens, cherry tomatoes, and balsamic vinaigrette.
- ***Dinner:*** Turkey chili with kidney beans and diced tomatoes, served with a side salad.

Continue this pattern for the remaining days, incorporating a variety of lean proteins, whole grains, fruits, vegetables, and healthy fats. Remember to avoid spicy, acidic, or fatty foods that may trigger gastritis symptoms.

Conclusion:

In "Super Easy Gastritis Diet and Recipes," we've embarked on a journey toward healing and nourishing our bodies. Throughout this book, we've explored the complexities of gastritis and discovered simple yet effective dietary strategies to alleviate symptoms and promote digestive health.

By incorporating gastritis-friendly foods and recipes into our daily routine, we've empowered ourselves to take control of our health and well-being. From soothing herbal teas to nutrient-rich meals, each recipe has been carefully crafted to support our bodies on the path to healing.

Remember, healing is a journey, not a destination. As we continue to prioritize our health and make mindful choices, we pave the way for a vibrant and thriving life. Let this book serve as a guide and companion on your journey toward optimal digestive health.

www.ingramcontent.com/pod-product-compliance
Lightning Source LLC
Chambersburg PA
CBHW050117230526
45470CB00004B/1879